Arachnoiditis

A Beginner's Quick Start Guide to Managing the Condition Through Diet and Other Natural Methods, With Sample Recipes

PATRICK MARSHWELL

Disclaimer

By reading this disclaimer, you are accepting the terms of the disclaimer in full. If you disagree with this disclaimer, please do not read the guide.

All of the content within this guide is provided for informational and educational purposes only, and should not be accepted as independent medical or other professional advice. The author is not a doctor, physician, nurse, mental health provider, or registered nutritionist/dietician. Therefore, using and reading this guide does not establish any form of a physician-patient relationship.

Always consult with a physician or another qualified health provider with any issues or questions you might have regarding any sort of medical condition. Do not ever disregard any qualified professional medical advice or delay seeking that advice because of anything you have read in this guide. The information in this guide is not intended to be any sort of medical advice and should not be used in lieu of any medical advice by a licensed and qualified medical professional.

The information in this guide has been compiled from a variety of known sources. However, the author cannot attest to or guarantee the accuracy of each source and thus should not be held liable for any errors or omissions.

Introduction

Arachnoiditis is an inflammation of the arachnoid, one of the three membranes that surround and protect the spinal cord and nerves. The arachnoid is a thin, spider web-like membrane that covers the central nervous system, which includes the brain and spinal cord. The other two membranes are called the dura mater and pia mater.

Arachnoiditis can be caused by several different things, including chemical irritation, bacterial or viral infection, direct spine damage, persistent spinal nerve compression, or consequences from spinal surgery. These conditions can inflame the arachnoid, which can lead to the formation of scar tissue and adhesions. These adhesions can bind spinal nerves, which can then cause chronic pain, numbness, tingling, stinging, and burning sensations in the lower back or legs. Arachnoiditis can also cause muscle cramps, jerks, and spasms.

In some cases, arachnoiditis can also lead to bladder, bowel, and sexual dysfunction. In severe cases, arachnoiditis can even cause lower-limb paralysis.

There is no cure for arachnoiditis, but there are treatments that can help manage the symptoms and improve quality of life.

In this quick start guide, we will discuss the following:

- What are the types of arachnoiditis?
- What are the symptoms of arachnoiditis?
- What causes arachnoiditis?
- What are its risk factors?
- When to see a doctor?
- How is arachnoiditis diagnosed?
- What are the treatments for arachnoiditis?
- Prognosis of arachnoiditis.
- Managing arachnoiditis through natural methods.

What are the foods to eat and avoid if you have arachnoiditis?

So, let's get started.

Table of Contents

WHAT ARE THE TYPES OF ARACHNOIDITIS

There are different forms of arachnoiditis.

Adhesive arachnoiditis: Adhesive arachnoiditis is a condition in which the layers of tissue that surround the brain and spinal cord become stuck together. This can cause chronic pain, inflammation, and nerve damage. Adhesive arachnoiditis is often caused by injections or surgery around the spine.

Arachnoiditis Ossificans: Arachnoiditis ossificans is a rare condition that results in the deterioration of the arachnoid, a membrane that surrounds and protects the spinal cord. The most common symptom of arachnoiditis ossificans is severe back pain, which can be debilitating. Other symptoms may include weakness, numbness, and tingling in the legs or arms. In some cases, arachnoiditis ossificans can cause paralysis.

Cerebral Arachnoiditis: Cerebral arachnoiditis is a type of arachnoiditis that specifically affects the brain. It can be caused by several different things, including infections, certain medical procedures, and head injuries. Symptoms of cerebral arachnoiditis include headaches, stiffness in the neck and shoulders, numbness or tingling in the arms and legs, dizziness, and problems with balance.

Hereditary Arachnoiditis: Hereditary arachnoiditis is a rare neurological disorder that is passed down through families. The disorder affects the arachnoid membrane, which is a layer of tissue that covers the brain and spinal cord. Hereditary arachnoiditis can cause a variety of symptoms, including chronic pain, seizures, and paralysis.

Neoplastic Arachnoiditis: Neoplastic arachnoiditis is a rare condition characterized by the growth of neoplasms, or tumors, in the arachnoid membrane. Neoplastic arachnoiditis can be caused by a variety of factors, including exposure to radiation, chemotherapy, and certain viruses.

Optochiasmatic Arachnoiditis: Optochiasmatic Arachnoiditis is an abnormal thickening of the optic nerve arachnoid. Optic chiasm connects the two optic nerves. This area can get arachnoiditis from tuberculosis or tapeworms. Optochiasmatic arachnoiditis is also linked to encephalitis.

Post Myelographic Arachnoiditis: Post Myelographic arachnoiditis is the more common form, and it is caused by the inflammatory reaction that occurs after a spinal myelogram. In this procedure, dye is injected into the spinal canal to allow the spine to be seen more clearly on an X-ray or CT scan. However, the dye can sometimes cause an inflammatory reaction that leads to arachnoiditis.

Rhinosinus Ogenic Cerebral Arachnoiditis: Rhinosinus Ogenic Cerebral Arachnoiditis (RCA) is a subtype of cerebral arachnoiditis that is linked with sinus inflammation (rhinosinusitis). RCA is a serious, chronic, and progressive neurological condition that can lead to severe disability and even death.

These different types of arachnoiditis can be caused by a variety of things. Some are more serious than others, and some may even be hereditary. Arachnoiditis is not always easy to diagnose because the symptoms can be similar to other conditions. That's why it's important to see a doctor if you think you might have this condition.

SYMPTOMS OF ARACHNOIDITIS

The symptoms of arachnoiditis can vary depending on the severity of the condition and which nerves are affected. However, common symptoms include:

Chronic pain: Chronic pain is the most common symptom of arachnoiditis, and can be described as achy, sharp, burning, or stinging. This type of pain is typically constant and can worsen with activity or movement.

Neurological deficits: Neurological deficits refer to problems with nerve function, such as numbness, weakness, and difficulty walking. These symptoms can vary in severity and may come and go over time. In some cases, arachnoiditis can lead to paralysis.

Involuntary Movements: One of the most distinctive symptoms of arachnoiditis is involuntary muscle movements, such as cramps, spasms, or jerking. These movements can be painful and may make it difficult to perform everyday activities. In some cases, the muscles may become so weak that they are unable to support the body.

Bladder dysfunction: One symptom of arachnoiditis is bladder dysfunction. The individual may find it difficult to control their bladder, and they may experience urinary retention or incontinence.

In some cases, the individual may also experience pelvic pain. The exact nature of the bladder dysfunction will depend on the underlying cause of the arachnoiditis. For example, if the condition is caused by an infection, the individual may experience frequent urination due to inflammation of the bladder. If the condition is caused by scarring of the nerves, the individual may lose the ability to empty their bladder.

Bowel dysfunction: One symptom of arachnoiditis is bowel dysfunction. This may manifest as either constipation or diarrhea and may be accompanied by bloating, cramping, or abdominal pain.

The exact cause of bowel dysfunction is not known, but it is thought to be related to the inflammation of the arachnoid membrane. This inflammation can damage nerve fibers that are responsible for regulating bowel function.

Sexual dysfunction: One symptom of Arachnoiditis that is not often talked about is sexual dysfunction. This can present itself in both men and women and can have a severely negative impact on quality of life. In men, Arachnoiditis can cause erectile dysfunction and loss of libido. In women, it can cause pain during intercourse, loss of libido, and difficulty achieving orgasm.

These symptoms can vary in severity from person to person. Some people may only experience mild discomfort, while others may have debilitating pain that prevents them from living a normal life. The symptoms can also come and go, or they may be constant. In some cases, the symptoms may even get worse over time.

If you think you may have arachnoiditis, it is important to see a doctor so that you can get an accurate diagnosis and start treatment as soon as possible. Early diagnosis and treatment are the best way to manage the symptoms of arachnoiditis and improve quality of life.

CAUSES OF ARACHNOIDITIS

Arachnoiditis is a rare condition that occurs when the arachnoid, one of the membranes that surround the nerves of the spinal cord, becomes inflamed. This inflammation can be caused by a variety of factors, including chemical irritation, infection, and physical trauma. In some cases, the exact cause of the inflammation is unknown.

Chemical irritation: Chemical irritation of the arachnoid is often seen in patients who have undergone spinal surgery. The chemicals used during surgery, such as anesthetics and disinfectants, can irritate the arachnoid and lead to inflammation.

Bacterial or viral infection: Bacterial or viral infections are another common cause of arachnoiditis. The bacteria that cause infections, such as tuberculosis and meningitis, can inflame the arachnoid and damage the nerves. In some cases, a virus can also lead to arachnoiditis.

Physical trauma: Physical trauma to the spine can also lead to arachnoiditis. A slip and fall, car accident, or another traumatic event can cause the membranes to become damaged and inflamed.

Persistent spinal nerve compression: This can happen if something, such as a tumor or herniated disc, puts pressure on the spinal nerves. This pressure can inflame the arachnoid and cause arachnoiditis.

Consequences from spinal surgery: In some cases, arachnoiditis can be a complication of spinal surgery. This is more likely to happen if surgery is performed near the spine or if multiple surgeries are performed.

These conditions can inflame the arachnoid, which can lead to the formation of scar tissue and adhesions. These adhesions can bind spinal nerves, which can then cause chronic pain, numbness, tingling, stinging, and burning sensations in the lower back or legs. Arachnoiditis can also cause muscle cramps, jerks, and spasms.

In some cases, arachnoiditis can also lead to bladder, bowel, and sexual dysfunction. In severe cases, arachnoiditis can even cause lower-limb paralysis.

RISK FACTORS FOR ARACHNOIDITIS

Arachnoiditis most commonly affects the lumbar region of the spine, but it can occur in the cervical and thoracic regions as well. The condition is more common in women than men, and typically affects people between the ages of 40 and 60.

Other several risk factors can increase your chances of developing arachnoiditis, including:

Previous spinal surgery or trauma: One of the risk factors for developing arachnoiditis is previous spinal surgery or trauma. This is because, when the spine is surgically manipulated or injured, there is a higher chance that the delicate arachnoid membrane will be damaged. Once this happens, inflammation and scarring can occur, leading to the development of arachnoiditis.

If you have had spinal surgery or trauma in the past, it is important to be aware of this risk factor and to monitor your health closely for signs of arachnoiditis.

Multiple spinal injections: When a needle is inserted into the spine, it can inadvertently damage the arachnoid, leading to inflammation. In addition, the injected material can also irritate the arachnoid, furthering the inflammatory process.

As a result, those who have had multiple spinal injections are at a higher risk of developing arachnoiditis. If you have had multiple spinal injections, it is important to be aware of this risk factor and to talk to your doctor about any symptoms you may be experiencing.

Bacterial or viral infection: One of the risk factors for developing arachnoiditis is a previous bacterial or viral infection. This is because the infection can inflame the arachnoid membrane, causing it to become irritated and scarred. The resulting scarring can lead to the formation of adhesions, which can stick the arachnoid membrane to the spinal cord or nerve roots.

In severe cases, the adhesions can cause the spinal cord or nerve roots to become twisted, leading to pain, numbness, and weakness. If you have had a bacterial or viral infection, it is important to monitor your symptoms and seek medical attention if you develop any new or worsening neurological symptoms.

Spinal tumors: One risk factor for developing arachnoiditis is having spinal tumors. While spinal tumors are not always cancerous, they can still cause a great deal of damage to the delicate tissues surrounding the spine.

In particular, they can put pressure on the nerves and blood vessels in the spine, leading to inflammation and pain. In addition, spinal tumors can also cause scar tissue to form around the nerve roots. This scar tissue can eventually lead to the development of arachnoiditis.

If you have been diagnosed with a spinal tumor, it is important to discuss your risks with your doctor so that you can take steps to prevent or delay the onset of this condition.

Herniated discs: One of the most common risk factors for developing arachnoiditis is a herniated disc. When a disc herniates, it puts pressure on the nerves in the spine, which can lead to inflammation and scarring of the delicate arachnoid membrane. This can cause severe pain, numbness, and weakness in the affected area.

In some cases, it can also lead to paralysis. If you have herniated discs, it is important to get treatment as soon as possible to reduce your risk of developing arachnoiditis. Treatment options include physical therapy, medication, and surgery.

WHEN TO SEE A DOCTOR?

If you are experiencing back pain, numbness, tingling, or other symptoms that might be associated with arachnoiditis, it is important to see a doctor so that you can get an accurate diagnosis and start treatment as soon as possible.

Furthermore, if you are at risk of developing arachnoiditis, it is important to talk to your doctor about steps you can take to prevent or delay the onset of this condition.

Arachnoiditis is a serious condition that can cause severe pain, disability, and even paralysis. However, with early diagnosis and treatment, many people with this condition can lead normal, active lives.

Diagnosis of Arachnoiditis

Arachnoiditis is typically diagnosed using a combination of medical history, physical examination, imaging tests, and nerve studies. No one test can definitively diagnose arachnoiditis. Your doctor will likely order a variety of tests to rule out other conditions with similar symptoms.

Medical history: A complete medical history is important for diagnosing arachnoiditis. Your doctor will ask about any previous spinal surgery or trauma, infections, tumors, herniated discs, and spinal injections. This information will help your doctor rule out other conditions and better understand your symptoms.

Physical examination: Your doctor will look for signs of tenderness, muscle spasms, and loss of sensation in the lower back or legs. If these signs are present, your doctor may order further tests to confirm the diagnosis. These tests may include imaging studies or a nerve conduction study.

Imaging tests: Your doctor will likely suspect arachnoiditis based on your symptoms and medical history. To confirm the diagnosis, your doctor may order one or more imaging tests. MRI and CT scans are both effective at visualizing the spine and identifying signs of arachnoiditis.

Nerve studies: One of the most common diagnostic tools for arachnoiditis is nerve studies, such as electromyography (EMG) or nerve conduction study (NCS). These tests help to assess the function of the nervous system and can often provide clues as to the underlying cause of the condition.

TREATMENT OF ARACHNOIDITIS

Treatment of arachnoiditis typically involves a combination of pain medication, physical therapy, and spinal injections. Surgery is rarely needed. Pain medication can help to relieve the pain associated with arachnoiditis. Physical therapy can help to stretch and strengthen the muscles surrounding the affected area. Spinal injections can help to reduce inflammation and pain. Surgery is only considered in cases where the pain is severe and other treatments have failed.

Pain medication: Arachnoiditis can cause severe pain, although pain medicine, such as opioids, can help alleviate some of the discomforts. Because of the potential for dependence and addiction, these medicines should only be taken when necessary.

Physical therapy: Physical therapy is one treatment option that can help to stretch and strengthen the muscles surrounding the affected area. This can help to reduce pain and improve the range of motion. In addition, physical therapy can help to prevent further damage to the nerves and improve function.

Spinal injections: Spinal injections, such as epidural steroid injections, can be used to reduce inflammation and pain. However, these injections should be used sparingly, as they can lead to side effects such as infection and nerve damage.

Surgery: Surgery is only considered in cases where the pain is severe and other treatments have failed. Surgery is typically used to decompress the nerves or fuse the vertebrae. In some cases, a spinal cord stimulator may be implanted to help block pain signals.

Many persons who have arachnoiditis can enjoy normal, active lives if they receive an accurate diagnosis and treatment as soon as possible.

ARACHNOIDITIS PROGNOSIS

The prognosis for arachnoiditis is generally good. Most people with arachnoiditis can manage their symptoms with conservative treatment. However, some people may experience chronic pain and disability.

Chronic Pain: Arachnoiditis is a potential source of ongoing pain. This pain could be sporadic or it could be chronic. Its severity might range from hardly noticeable to completely incapacitating. The presence of persistent pain can have a detrimental effect on one's quality of life.

Disability: There is a possibility of incapacity for some patients who have arachnoiditis. This may be because of the persistent pain that comes along with the illness. A person's quality of life may suffer as a result of their disability.

Quality of life: Arachnoiditis has the potential to have a detrimental effect on one's quality of life. The persistent pain and incapacity that are often linked with the disorder might make it challenging to carry out activities of daily living.

MANAGING ARACHNOIDITIS THROUGH NATURAL METHODS

Physical Therapy: One of the most important things you can do to manage arachnoiditis is to keep your back and spine as healthy as possible. Physical therapy can help to stretch and strengthen the muscles surrounding the affected area. This can help to reduce pain and improve the range of motion.

Exercise: Exercise is important for maintaining a healthy back and spine. It can help to reduce the pain associated with arachnoiditis. Exercise can also help to improve the range of motion.

Proper posture: Maintaining proper posture can help to reduce the pain associated with arachnoiditis. Proper posture helps to take the pressure off of the affected area.

Hot and cold therapy: Applying heat or ice to the affected area can help to reduce pain. Heat can help to increase blood flow to the area and relax the muscles. Ice can help to reduce inflammation.

Massage: Massage can help to reduce pain and improve circulation. Massage can also help to relax the muscles.

Acupuncture: Acupuncture is a traditional Chinese medicine technique that involves the insertion of needles into the skin. Acupuncture can help to reduce pain and improve circulation.

Yoga: Yoga can help to improve flexibility and strength. Yoga can also help to relax the mind and body.

Meditation: Meditation can help to relax the mind and body. Meditation can also help to improve focus and concentration.

Arachnoiditis is a condition that causes inflammation of the arachnoid membrane, which is a layer of tissue that surrounds the spinal cord. Arachnoiditis can cause severe pain, muscle weakness, numbness, and paralysis. There is no cure for arachnoiditis, but there are treatments that can help to manage the pain and other symptoms associated with the condition. Treatment typically focuses on relieving pain and other symptoms and preventing further damage to the spinal cord.

Physical therapy, exercise, and proper posture can all help to reduce pain and improve the range of motion. Hot and cold therapy, massage, acupuncture, yoga, and meditation can all help to reduce pain and improve circulation. Surgery is only considered in cases where the pain is severe and other treatments have failed.

MANAGING ARACHNOIDITIS THROUGH DIET

Arachnoiditis is a debilitating condition that can cause chronic pain, numbness, and weakness. While there is no cure for arachnoiditis, making certain dietary choices can help manage the symptoms and improve your quality of life.

Foods to Eat

Fiber-rich diet: A diet rich in fiber may help to reduce inflammation and pain associated with arachnoiditis. Fiber-rich foods include fruits, vegetables, whole grains, and legumes. Fruits and vegetables are especially good sources of soluble fiber, which has been shown to help reduce inflammation. Including more fiber-rich foods in your diet may help to reduce the symptoms of arachnoiditis.

Antioxidant-rich diet: The nervous system is susceptible to damage from free radicals. Free radicals are unstable molecules that cause cell damage, and they have been linked to several degenerative diseases. Antioxidants are believed to help protect cells from free radical damage, and a diet rich in antioxidants may help to reduce the risk of developing degenerative diseases. Dark leafy greens, berries, nuts, and seeds are all excellent sources of antioxidants.

Omega-3 fatty acids: Omega-3 fatty acids may help to reduce pain and inflammation. Omega-3 fatty acids are found in fish, flaxseeds, chia seeds, and other food sources. They have been shown to have anti-inflammatory properties, which may help to reduce the symptoms of arachnoiditis. In addition, omega-3 fatty acids can also help to improve joint function and reduce stiffness.

Foods to Avoid

While certain foods can help to reduce pain and inflammation, there are also some foods that you should avoid if you have arachnoiditis.

Nightshade vegetables: Nightshade vegetables can increase inflammation and contribute to the development of arachnoiditis. Nightshade vegetables, such as tomatoes, potatoes, peppers, and eggplants, contain compounds called alkaloids. These alkaloids can increase inflammation and cause pain, numbness, and tingling in the extremities.

In addition, nightshade vegetables are often high in sugar and carbohydrates, which can also contribute to inflammation.

Dairy products: Inflammation is a response by the body to infection, irritation, or injury. The symptoms of inflammation include pain, redness, swelling, and heat. Dairy products are a common source of inflammation for many people. Dairy products can contain high levels of saturated fat, which can increase inflammation and pain.

In addition, dairy products can contain hormones and other growth factors that can promote inflammation. For these reasons, people who suffer from arachnoiditis may need to avoid dairy products.

Sugar: Sugar can have many negative effects on the body, including inflammation and pain. Inflammation is a normal response to injury or infection, but it can become chronic if left unchecked. Sugar promotes inflammation by binding to inflammatory proteins called kinases.

Alcohol: Alcohol consumption can lead to increased inflammation and pain. Alcohol is a diuretic, which causes the body to lose fluids and become dehydrated. Dehydration can cause the body to produce fewer natural painkilling substances, called endorphins. In addition, alcohol consumption can interfere with the functioning of immune cells, leading to increased inflammation.

In addition, alcohol can interfere with the body's ability to absorb nutrients, which can also lead to increased pain. While moderate alcohol consumption is generally considered safe, it is important to be aware of the potential risks associated with excessive drinking.

Caffeine: Caffeine is a stimulant that is widely consumed for its ability to improve alertness and wakefulness. However, caffeine can also have several undesirable effects, particularly in large doses. One of the most significant problems associated with caffeine consumption is increased inflammation.

In addition, caffeine can also worsen pain by interfering with the body's natural pain-relieving mechanisms. For these reasons, it is important to limit caffeine intake, particularly if you are already suffering from inflammation or pain.

By following a healthy diet and avoiding foods that can trigger inflammation, you can help to reduce pain and other symptoms associated with arachnoiditis.

SAMPLE RECIPES

Baked Salmon

Ingredients:

- 2 salmon filets
- 6 cups of fresh spinach
- 2 tsp. coconut oil
- 1/4 tsp. garlic powder
- 1/4 tsp. turmeric
- 3 large cloves of garlic
- lemon juice
- salt
- pepper

Instructions:

1. Preheat the oven to 400°F.
2. Line a baking dish with parchment paper.
3. Marinate salmon filets in lemon juice, coconut oil, garlic powder, turmeric, salt, and pepper.
4. Let it sit for a few minutes. This may also be done the night before to help the juices and flavor get into the salmon.

5. Once the oven is ready, bake the salmon for 15 minutes.
6. Cook some of the garlic in a pan with coconut oil.
7. Add spinach and cook until ready. Season with salt and pepper to taste.
8. Take salmon out of the oven and put spinach beside it.
9. Serve and enjoy.

Baked Salmon with Asparagus

Ingredients:

- 1.5 lbs. wild salmon
- 2 tbsp. olive oil
- 3 cloves garlic, minced
- 1 tsp. dried oregano
- pepper
- sea salt
- 1 bunch fresh asparagus
- 1/2 cup cucumber
- 1/2 cup olives
- 1 whole lemon

Instructions:

1. Preheat the oven to 400°F.
2. Use parchment paper to line a baking sheet. Set aside.
3. Mix oil, oregano, salt, garlic, and pepper in a bowl.
4. Pour seasoning mix over the salmon and coat the entire fish.
5. Layer the salmon on the baking sheet.

6. Place trimmed asparagus on the sheet pan next to the salmon.
7. Squeeze fresh lemon juice and place remaining lemon slices on the sheet pan. Bake for 20 minutes.
8. When the salmon is done, serve with a scoop of olive & feta salad over the salmon or on the side and serve.

Tuna and Veggies Wrap

Ingredients:

- 1 canned tuna
- 2 pcs. whole-grain tortillas
- 1 cup cucumber, sliced
- 1 tbsp. low-fat Italian dressing
- 1 cup carrots, julienned

Instructions:

1. Put the dressing and tuna in a bowl and mix well.
2. Arrange half of the mixture on one of the tortillas. Add half the amount of each vegetable and wrap.
3. Do the same to the remaining tortilla.

Fresh Asparagus Salad

Ingredients:

- 1/3 cup of hazelnuts
- 4 cups arugula
- 1 tsp. ground pepper

- 4 tsp. lemon juice
- 2 tbsp. sea salt
- virgin olive oil
- 2 lbs. asparagus

Instructions:

1. Preheat the oven to 400°F.
2. Place hazelnuts on a baking tray with parchment paper. Place in the oven for 7 minutes.
3. Transfer hazelnuts to a plate. Optionally, to remove the skins, wrap the nuts in a towel and rub them vigorously.
4. Chop hazelnuts coarsely.
5. Remove the hard ends of the asparagus.
6. Place the stalks on the baking sheet you've used for the hazelnuts. Sprinkle 1 tbsp. olive oil and 1/2 tsp. of salt.
7. Bake for 8 minutes.
8. In a mixing bowl, combine pepper, salt, olive oil, and lemon juice. Mix well.
9. Place the arugula in a medium bowl. Drizzle half of the dressing over the veggies. Toss until everything is well coated.
10. Place arugula onto a platter.
11. Arrange asparagus on top. Sprinkle peeled hazelnuts on top.

Arugula and Mushroom Salad

Ingredients:

- 5 oz. arugula washed

- 1 lb. fresh mushrooms
- 1/4 tsp. shoyu
- 1/2 red onion
- 1 tbsp. olive oil
- 1 tbsp. mirin

For tofu cheese:

- 1/8 cup umeboshi vinegar
- 1/2 firm tofu

Instructions:

1. In a bowl, add the rinsed tofu. Crumble and pour in vinegar.
2. In a separate bowl add shoyu, red onions, salt, olive oil, and mirin. 3. Mix to combine.
3. Add in the arugula and toss to combine with the dressing.
4. Serve and enjoy.

Asian Zucchini Salad

Ingredients:

- 1 medium zucchini, sliced thinly into spirals
- 1/3 cup rice vinegar
- 3/4 cup avocado oil
- 1 cup sunflower seeds, shells removed
- 1 lb. cabbage, shredded
- 1 tsp. stevia drops

- 1 cup almonds, sliced

Instructions:

1. Cut the zucchini spirals into smaller parts. Set aside.
2. Put almonds, sunflower seeds, and cabbage in a large bowl. Combine the ingredients well.
3. Add zucchini to the mixture.
4. In a small bowl, mix vinegar, stevia, and oil using a whisk or fork.
5. Pour the vinegar mixture all over the zucchini mixture. Toss well. Make sure everything is covered with the dressing.
6. Refrigerate for 2 hours before serving.

Chickpea Curry

Ingredients:

- 2 tbsp. vegetable oil
- 1 cup of fresh cilantro, chopped finely
- 2 onions, minced
- 2 15-oz. cans of garbanzo beans
- 2 cloves minced garlic
- 1 tsp. ground turmeric
- 2 tsp. fresh ginger root, chopped finely
- 1 tsp. black pepper
- 6 whole cloves of garlic
- salt
- 2 cinnamon sticks, crushed
- 1 tsp. ground coriander

- 1 tsp. ground cumin

Instructions:

1. Heat oil in a frying pan over medium heat.
2. Sauté onion until they turn tender.
3. Stir in ginger, garlic, coriander, cinnamon, cumin, cayenne, and turmeric. Cook them for a minute while stirring constantly.
4. Mix garbanzo beans and their liquid into the mixture.
5. Continue cooking while stirring frequently.
6. Remove from heat. Stir in cilantro.
7. Serve immediately.

Roasted Pumpkin and Brussel Sprouts

Ingredients:

- 3 lb. pie pumpkin, peeled and cut into ¾-inch cubes
- 1 lb. fresh Brussels sprouts, trimmed and halved lengthwise
- 1 tsp. sea salt
- 1/2 tsp. coarsely ground pepper
- 1/3 cup olive oil
- 2 tbsp. balsamic vinegar
- 2 tbsp. minced fresh parsley
- 4 garlic cloves, thinly sliced

Instructions:

1. Preheat the oven to 400°F.
2. Combine Brussels sprouts, garlic, and pumpkin in a bowl.
3. Whisk oil, vinegar, salt, and pepper in a separate bowl.
4. Drizzle the mixture over the vegetables. Toss gently.
5. Pour the coated vegetables onto a greased baking pan.
6. Roast until tender, about 35-40 minutes. Stir once.
7. Sprinkle with parsley upon serving.

Vegetable Casserole Medley

Ingredients:

- 1 cup or jar of squash sauce
- 1 zucchini and/or squash, sliced
- 1 small onion, chopped
- 1 bag fresh or frozen cauliflower
- 1 sleeve saltines, crushed
- salt
- white pepper

Instructions:

1. Add some cooking spray to a dish
2. Add one layer of sliced zucchini or sliced zucchini and squash.
3. Add the onions and cauliflower florets over zucchini
4. Pour sauce over all of the vegetable ingredients
5. Add the saltines.
6. Place this inside the oven. Bake at 370°F for 50 minutes.
7. Do a fork test by poking through the vegetables.

8. Bake for another 20 minutes if you want tender vegetables.

Tuna Salad

Ingredients:

- 1/2 cup pecans
- 1 cup chicken breast, steamed and cubed
- 1 cup tuna in oil
- salt, to taste
- pepper, to taste

Instructions:

1. Mix all ingredients in a large bowl.
2. Add a dash of salt and pepper to taste.
3. Chill for at least an hour before serving.

Conclusion

Arachnoiditis is a painful condition that can cause chronic pain, numbness, and weakness. While there is no cure for arachnoiditis, making certain dietary choices can help manage the symptoms and improve your quality of life.

A diet rich in fiber, antioxidants, and omega-3 fatty acids can help to reduce inflammation and pain. Nightshade vegetables, dairy products, sugar, alcohol, and caffeine can all increase inflammation and pain.

If you've had an epidural steroid injection or spinal anesthesia, it's important to see your doctor for an annual physical so that any early signs of arachnoiditis can be detected and treated.

FAQ About Arachnoiditis

1. What is arachnoiditis?

Arachnoiditis is a condition that affects the nerves in the spinal cord. The symptoms of arachnoiditis can include chronic pain, numbness, and weakness. There is no cure for arachnoiditis, but there are treatments that can help to manage the symptoms.

2. What causes arachnoiditis?

Arachnoiditis can be caused by several different things, including epidural steroid injections, spinal anesthesia, surgery, and infections.

3. How is arachnoiditis diagnosed?

Arachnoiditis is usually diagnosed through a combination of a physical examination, imaging tests, and nerve studies.

4. What are the treatments for arachnoiditis?

There is no cure for arachnoiditis, but there are treatments that can help to manage the symptoms. These treatments include pain medication, physical therapy, and surgery.

5. Can arachnoiditis be prevented?

There is no sure way to prevent arachnoiditis, but there are some things that you can do to lower your risk. If you've had an epidural steroid injection or spinal anesthesia, it's important to see your doctor for an annual physical so that any early signs of arachnoiditis can be detected and treated.

6. How to manage arachnoiditis through a natural method?

There is no cure for arachnoiditis, but there are treatments that can help to manage the symptoms. These treatments include pain medication, physical therapy, and surgery. Some people also find relief by making dietary changes, such as eating a diet rich in fiber, antioxidants, and omega-3 fatty acids. Nightshade vegetables, dairy products, sugar, alcohol, and caffeine can all increase inflammation and pain.

7. What is the prognosis for arachnoiditis?

The prognosis for arachnoiditis is generally good, but the condition can cause chronic pain and disability. There is no cure for arachnoiditis, but there are treatments that can help to manage the symptoms.

References

Arachnoiditis | National Institute of Neurological Disorders and stroke. (n.d.). Retrieved October 13, 2022, from https://www.ninds.nih.gov/health-information/disorders/arachnoiditis.

Arachnoiditis: Symptoms, Types, Causes, and Treatment. (2018, February 2). https://www.medicalnewstoday.com/articles/320811.

Arachnoiditis: What It Is, Causes, Symptoms & Treatment. (n.d.). Cleveland Clinic. Retrieved October 13, 2022, from https://my.clevelandclinic.org/health/diseases/12062-arachnoiditis.

Australia, N. T. P. (n.d.). Natural treatments for arachnoiditis | treating arachnoiditis naturally | naturaltherapypages. Com. Au. Natural Therapy Pages. Retrieved October 13, 2022, from https://www.naturaltherapypages.com.au/article/natural-treatments-for-arachnoiditis.

Home. (n.d.). Retrieved October 13, 2022, from https://arachnoiditis.co.uk/.

www.ingramcontent.com/pod-product-compliance
Lightning Source LLC
Chambersburg PA
CBHW050621160726
48003CB00003B/1282